WEIGHT LOSS SMOOTHIES FOR SENIORS

50 Recipes to Rejuvenate Your Health and Shed Pounds

DR. JOSEPHINE W. PACK

TABLE OF CONTENTS

Mr. and Mrs. Ramsey, a lively elderly couple, had always shared an active lifestyle. As they entered their golden years, however, they noted a steady rise in their weight, which started to impede their movement and general well-being. Concerned about their health, they set out to discover a remedy that would help them to lose the weight and restore their vigor. While wandering at a local bookshop, they came upon a book that piqued their interest: "Weight Loss Smoothies for Seniors." They decided to give it a go since the title piqued their interest. They had no idea that this book would become a guiding light for them on their weight reduction quest.

Mr. and Mrs. Ramsey uncovered a treasure mine of healthful smoothie recipes made exclusively for seniors inside its pages. Each dish included a range of fruits, vegetables, and healthful components that encouraged not just weight reduction but also general health and life. They were so excited about the potential that they immediately began including these smoothies into their regular regimen. The results were fantastic. They saw an increase in their energy levels, a decrease in their appetites for unhealthy foods, and, most significantly, a reduction in their waistlines. As they continued to read the book, they discovered useful information on portion management, mindful eating, and age-appropriate exercise regimens. Armed with this newfound information, they adopted a holistic approach to their health, radically altering their lives.

Mr. and Mrs. Ramsey became role models for their peers, sharing their weight reduction success story and the book's vital ideas with their community's senior citizens. They became live evidence that age was not an impediment to reaching one's health objectives. Mr. and Mrs. Ramsey not only lost weight but also recovered their passion for life thanks to the book's counsel and their steadfast devotion. Their voyage of discovery with "Weight Loss Smoothies for Seniors" had been genuinely transforming, reaffirming the power of information, dedication, and good choices in their life.

CHAPTER 1. Weight Loss Smoothies in Brief

Smoothies for weight reduction have grown in popularity in recent years as a handy and efficient approach to reduce unwanted pounds. These healthy drinks are often produced by combining a variety of fruits, vegetables, and other ingredients to provide a tasty and healthy meal replacement alternative. Weight loss smoothies are not only tasty but also high in critical nutrients, making them a fantastic alternative for anyone looking to lose weight.

Smoothies Are Important for Seniors

Smoothies are very important for seniors who want to maintain their weight successfully. Our bodies change as we age, which may affect metabolism, digestion, and total nutritional absorption. Furthermore, keeping a healthy weight is becoming increasingly important in the prevention and management of age-related health disorders such as diabetes, heart disease, and joint difficulties. Smoothies are an easy and fun method for seniors to have a nutrient-dense meal while keeping their calorie consumption under control.

CHAPTER 2. Understanding Seniors Weight Loss Smoothies

Factors Influencing Seniors Weight Loss

Weight loss in seniors may be influenced by a variety of variables, including muscle mass loss, hormonal changes, a slower metabolism, and age-related health issues. These characteristics may make it more difficult for seniors to lose weight with typical dieting strategies. Weight loss smoothies, on the other hand, may give a practical option by providing balanced nutrients, inducing satiety, and supporting healthy weight control.

Weight Loss Smoothie Advantages for Seniors

Weight reduction smoothies provide various advantages for seniors who are trying to lose weight. **Here are some significant benefits:**

a)Nutrient Density:
Smoothies may be high in nutrients such as vitamins, minerals, antioxidants, and fiber. This nutritional density ensures that seniors obtain a

diverse spectrum of critical nutrients while maintaining a healthy calorie consumption.

b) Hydration:

Many seniors fail to drink enough fluids, which may contribute to dehydration. Weight reduction smoothies, which are often prepared with water, milk, or coconut water as a basis, may help seniors remain hydrated while also providing a tasty and pleasant beverage.

c) Digestive Wellness:

Seniors' digestion and nutrition absorption might be affected by age-related changes. Smoothies, particularly those containing fiber-rich foods such as fruits, vegetables, and whole grains, may help with digestive health, constipation relief, and nutritional absorption.

d) Meal Substitution:

Weight loss smoothies may be useful meal alternatives for seniors, enabling them to regulate their portion sizes and calorie consumption. They are simple to make, can be modified to individual tastes, and can be enjoyed on the move, making them an appealing alternative for seniors who lead busy lives.

e) Controlling Hunger and Satiety:
Smoothies, owing to their high fiber and protein content, may offer a sensation of fullness and satisfaction. This may assist seniors in managing food urges and avoiding overeating, resulting in good weight reduction.

Finally, weight loss smoothies are a great tool for seniors who want to efficiently control their weight. Smoothies may help seniors who are trying to lose weight live a better and more active lifestyle by delivering nutrient-dense meals, encouraging hydration, supporting digestion, and assisting in appetite management.

CHAPTER 3. Green Detox Smoothie

Ingredients:

Spinach, cucumber, green apple, celery, lemon juice, and water make up the Green Detox Smoothie.

Preparation:

All items should be combined and blended together smoothly.

Make sure you wash all the necessary ingredients.

Berry Blast Smoothie

Ingredients:

Strawberries, blueberries, and raspberries, almond milk, Greek yogurt, and chia seeds.

Preparation:

All items should be combined and blended together smoothly.

Make sure you wash all the necessary ingredients.

Tropical Delight Smoothie

Ingredients:

pineapple, mango, banana, coconut water, and spinach.

Preparation:

All items should be washed, combined and blended together smoothly.

Make sure you wash all the necessary ingredients.

Creamy Avocado Smoothie

Ingredients:

Avocado, almond milk, banana, spinach, and honey are the ingredients for this creamy avocado smoothie.

Preparation:

All items should be washed, combined and blended together smoothly.

Make sure you wash all the necessary ingredients.

Apple Cinnamon Smoothie

Ingredients:

Apple, almond milk, Greek yogurt, cinnamon, and ice.

Preparation:

All items should be combined and blended together smoothly.

Make sure you wash all the necessary ingredients.

Chocolate Banana Smoothie

Ingredients:

Banana, almond milk, chocolate powder, and honey.

Preparation:

All items should be combined and blended together smoothly.

Make sure you wash all the necessary ingredients.

CHAPTER 4. Citrus Boost Smoothie

Ingredients:
Orange, grapefruit, lemon, Greek yogurt, and honey.

Preparation:
All items should be combined and blended together smoothly.
Make sure you wash all the necessary ingredients.

Smoothie with Mixed Vegetables

Ingredients:
Carrots, tomatoes, cucumber, spinach, ginger, and water.

Preparation:
All items should be combined and blended together smoothly.
Make sure you wash all the necessary ingredients.

Peanut Butter Banana Smoothie

Ingredients:
Banana, almond milk, peanut butter, chia seeds

Preparation:

All items should be combined and blended together smoothly.

Make sure you wash all the necessary ingredients.

Pomegranate Berry Smoothie

Ingredients:

Pomegranate seeds, mixed berries, almond milk, and Greek yogurt are the ingredients for this smoothie.

Preparation:

All items should be combined and blended together smoothly.

Make sure you wash all the necessary ingredients.

Smoothie with Spinach and Mango

Ingredients:

Spinach, mango, coconut water, Greek yogurt, and honey.

Preparation:

All items should be combined and blended together smoothly.

Make sure you wash all the necessary ingredients.

Kiwi Lime Smoothie

Ingredients:
kiwi, lime juice, almond milk, spinach, and honey.

Preparation:
All items should be combined and blended together smoothly.
Make sure you wash all the necessary ingredients.

CHAPTER 5. Blueberry Almond Smoothie

Ingredients:

Blueberries, almond milk, almond butter, and Greek yogurt.

Preparation:

All items should be combined and blended together smoothly.

Make sure you wash all the necessary ingredients.

Watermelon Mint Smoothie

Ingredients:

Watermelon, mint leaves, coconut water, lime juice, and honey are the ingredients in this smoothie.

Preparation:

All items should be combined and blended together smoothly.

Make sure you wash all the necessary ingredients.

Pineapple Ginger Smoothie

Ingredients:

Pineapple, ginger, almond milk, Greek yogurt, and honey are the ingredients for this smoothie.

Preparation:

All items should be combined and blended together smoothly.

Make sure you wash all the necessary ingredients.

Mango Coconut Smoothie

Ingredients:

Mango, coconut milk, Greek yogurt, and chia seeds.

Preparation:

All items should be combined and blended together smoothly.

Make sure you wash all the necessary ingredients.

Raspberry Banana Smoothie

Ingredients:

Raspberries, banana, almond milk, Greek yogurt, and honey are the ingredients for this smoothie.

Preparation:

All items should be combined and blended together smoothly.

Make sure you wash all the necessary ingredients.

CHAPTER 6. Kale and Apple Smoothie

Ingredients:

Kale, apple, almond milk, Greek yogurt, and honey are the ingredients for this smoothie.

Preparation:

All items should be combined and blended together smoothly.

Make sure you wash all the necessary ingredients.

Cherry Vanilla Smoothie

Ingredients:

Cherries, almond milk, vanilla extract, Greek yogurt, and honey make up the Cherry Vanilla Smoothie.

Preparation:

All items should be combined and blended together smoothly.

Make sure you wash all the necessary ingredients.

Smoothie with Beets and Carrots

Ingredients:

Beets, carrots, orange juice, ginger, and honey.

Preparation:

All items should be combined and blended together smoothly.

Make sure you wash all the necessary ingredients.

Papaya Banana Smoothie

Ingredients:

Papaya, banana, coconut water, Greek yogurt, chia seeds.

Preparation:

All items should be combined and blended together smoothly.

Make sure you wash all the necessary ingredients.

Almond Joy Smoothie

Ingredients:

Almond milk, chocolate powder, almond butter, coconut flakes, and honey are the ingredients.

Preparation:

All items should be combined and blended together smoothly.

Make sure you wash all the necessary ingredients.

Ingredients:

Peaches, spinach, almond milk, Greek yogurt, and honey.

Preparation:

All items should be combined and blended together smoothly.

Make sure you wash all the necessary ingredients.

Carrot Cake Smoothie

Ingredients:

Carrots, almond milk, cinnamon, vanilla extract, and honey are the ingredients for this smoothie.

Preparation:

All items should be combined and blended together smoothly.

Make sure you wash all the necessary ingredients.

Mango Ginger Smoothie

Ingredients:

Mango, ginger, almond milk, Greek yogurt, and honey are the ingredients for this smoothie.

Preparation:

All items should be combined and blended together smoothly.

Make sure you wash all the necessary ingredients.

Cucumber Mint Smoothie

Ingredients:

Cucumber, mint leaves, Greek yogurt, honey, and water are the ingredients.

Preparation:

All items should be combined and blended together smoothly.

Make sure you wash all the necessary ingredients.

Strawberry Basil Smoothie

Ingredients:

Strawberries, basil leaves, almond milk, Greek yogurt, and honey are the ingredients for this smoothie.

Preparation:

All items should be combined and blended together smoothly.

Make sure you wash all the necessary ingredients.

CHAPTER 8. Pumpkin Spice Smoothie

Ingredients:

Pumpkin puree, almond milk, cinnamon, nutmeg, and honey.

Preparation:

All items should be combined and blended together smoothly.

Make sure you wash all the necessary ingredients.

Blueberry Spinach Smoothie

Ingredients:

Blueberries, spinach, almond milk, Greek yogurt, and honey are the ingredients for this smoothie.

Preparation:

All items should be combined and blended together smoothly.

Make sure you wash all the necessary ingredients.

Ginger Turmeric Smoothie

Ingredients:

Ginger, turmeric, pineapple, almond milk, and honey.

Preparation:

All items should be combined and blended together smoothly.

Make sure you wash all the necessary ingredients.

Smoothie with Matcha Green Tea

Ingredients:

Matcha powder, almond milk, banana, spinach, and honey.

Preparation:

All items should be combined and blended together smoothly.

Make sure you wash all the necessary ingredients.

Orange Carrot Ginger Smoothie

Ingredients:

Carrots, orange juice, ginger, Greek yogurt, and honey are the ingredients for this smoothie.

Preparation:

All items should be combined and blended together smoothly.

Make sure you wash all the necessary ingredients.

CHAPTER 9. Peanut Butter Chocolate Smoothie

Ingredients:
Almond milk, chocolate powder, peanut butter, banana, and honey are the ingredients in the Peanut Butter Chocolate Smoothie.

Preparation:
All items should be combined and blended together smoothly.
Make sure you wash all the necessary ingredients.

Cherry Almond Smoothie

Ingredients:
Cherries, almond milk, almond butter, Greek yogurt, and honey make up the Cherry Almond Smoothie.

Preparation:
All items should be combined and blended together smoothly.
Make sure you wash all the necessary ingredients.

Coconut Mango Lime Smoothie

Ingredients:

Mango, coconut milk, lime juice, spinach, and honey are the ingredients in this Coconut Mango Lime Smoothie.

Preparation:

All items should be combined and blended together smoothly.
Make sure you wash all the necessary ingredients.

Raspberry Coconut Chia Smoothie

Ingredients:

Raspberries, coconut milk, chia seeds, Greek yogurt, and honey are the ingredients in this smoothie.

Preparation:

All items should be combined and blended together Smoothly.
Make sure you wash all the necessary ingredients.

Vanilla Berry Protein Smoothie

Ingredients:

Mixed berries, almond milk, vanilla protein powder, spinach, and honey.

Preparation:

All items should be combined and blended together Smoothly.

Make sure you wash all the necessary ingredients.

Peach Oatmeal Smoothie

Ingredients:

Peaches, almond milk, rolled oats, Greek yogurt, and honey.

Preparation:

All items should be combined and blended together Smoothly.

Make sure you wash all the necessary ingredients.

CHAPTER 10. Green Tea Berry Smoothie

Ingredients:

Green tea, mixed berries, spinach, Greek yogurt, and honey are the ingredients in this smoothie.

Preparation:

All items should be combined and blended together Smoothly.

Make green tea and set it aside to cool. Make sure you wash all the necessary ingredients.

Almond Cherry Protein Smoothie

Ingredients:

Almond milk, cherries, almond butter, vanilla protein powder, and honey are the ingredients in this smoothie.

Preparation:

All items should be combined and blended together Smoothly.

Make sure you wash all the necessary ingredients.

Mango Mint Lime Smoothie

Ingredients:

Mango, mint leaves, lime juice, coconut water, and spinach are the ingredients for this smoothie.

Preparation:
All items should be combined and blended together Smoothly.
Make sure you wash all the necessary ingredients.

Watermelon Berry Smoothie

Ingredients:
Watermelon, mixed berries, coconut water, Greek yogurt, and honey are the ingredients in this smoothie.

Preparation:
All items should be combined and blended together Smoothly.
Make sure you wash all the necessary ingredients.

Pineapple Coconut Green Smoothie

Ingredients:

Pineapple, coconut milk, spinach, chia seeds, and honey are the ingredients in this smoothie.

Preparation:

All items should be combined and blended together Smoothly.

Make sure you wash all the necessary ingredients.

Blueberry Almond Chia Smoothie

Ingredients:

Blueberries, almond milk, chia seeds, almond butter, and honey are the ingredients in this smoothie.

Preparation:

All items should be combined and blended together Smoothly.

Make sure you wash all the necessary ingredients.

CHAPTER 11. Spinach Banana Protein Smoothie

Ingredients:

Spinach, banana, almond milk, vanilla protein powder, and honey are the ingredients in this smoothie.

Preparation:

All items should be combined and blended together Smoothly.

Make sure you wash all the necessary ingredients.

Mango Turmeric Smoothie

Ingredients:

Mango, turmeric, almond milk, Greek yogurt, and honey are the ingredients for this smoothie.

Preparation:

All itcms should bc combined and blended together Smoothly.

Make sure you wash all the necessary ingredients.

Avocado Berry Smoothie

Ingredients:

Avocado, mixed berries, almond milk, Greek yogurt, and honey are the ingredients.

Preparation:

All items should be combined and blended together Smoothly.

Make sure you wash all the necessary ingredients.

Peach Ginger Green Smoothie

Ingredients:

Peaches, ginger, spinach, coconut water, and honey are the ingredients in this smoothie.

Preparation:

All items should be combined and blended together Smoothly.

Make sure you wash all the necessary ingredients.

Chocolate Cherry Protein Smoothie

Ingredients:

Almond milk, cherries, cocoa powder, chocolate protein powder, and honey are the ingredients for this Chocolate Cherry Protein Smoothie.

Preparation:

All items should be combined and blended together Smoothly.

Make sure you wash all the necessary ingredients.

Pineapple Basil Smoothie

Ingredients:

Pineapple, basil leaves, coconut water, Greek yogurt, and honey are the ingredients in this smoothie.

Preparation:

All items should be combined and blended together Smoothly.

Make sure you wash all the necessary ingredients.

Enjoy these smoothie recipes for a healthy and refreshing weight reduction journey!

In conclusion, "Weight Loss Smoothies for Seniors" is a useful resource for older persons interested in embarking on a healthy and productive weight reduction path. The book acknowledges the special requirements and concerns that elders confront and provides practical answers in the shape of delectable smoothie recipes. Throughout the book, the author stresses the significance of nutrition and the advantages of include smoothies in a senior's diet. The book guarantees that the recipes supply the essential vitamins, minerals, and antioxidants by concentrating on complete, nutrient-dense foods.

Furthermore, "Weight Loss Smoothies for Seniors" considers probable challenges that older people may have, such as reduced appetite or special dietary limitations. It provides versatile recipes that may be readily adapted to suit a variety of tastes and dietary requirements. What distinguishes this book is its focus on the total well-being of elders. It promotes higher energy levels, better digestion, and improved cognitive function in addition to weight reduction. It acknowledges that losing weight is just one part of living a healthy and fulfilled life in your older years.

Finally, "Weight Loss Smoothies for Seniors" is a thorough guide for older persons looking for a healthy and pleasurable approach to lose weight. This book inspires seniors to take charge of their health and enjoy a bright and active lifestyle by combining nutritional understanding with delectable recipes.

Dear Respected Customers,

We'd like to offer our heartfelt appreciation for selecting our book and entrusting us with your time. Your steadfast support and insightful comments mean everything to us. We sincerely appreciate your aid in submitting an honest evaluation as we always endeavor to enhance our work and produce engaging information. Your evaluations are very valuable not just to us as writers, but also to future readers looking for information. We really respect your views and comments, whether you felt our book was amazing or feel there were flaws. Your feedback is an ongoing source of inspiration for us to develop tales that are truly meaningful to you.

We would appreciate it if you could take a few seconds to share your Amazon review, as your comments have the potential to dramatically affect the success and reach of our book, helping it to reach a bigger audience. Your review does not have to be long or complicated. Simply giving your honest opinions, emphasizing areas that connected with you, or underlining notable components would be quite beneficial.

Once again, we express our deepest appreciation for being a part of our literary journey. Your ongoing support and participation are critical to us. We look forward to reading your evaluations and developing with you.

Best regards,

www.ingramcontent.com/pod-product-compliance
Lightning Source LLC
Chambersburg PA
CBHW070232260726
48658CB00006BA/2284